the unfiltered companion guide

to

This Wasn't in the Pamphlet

mary van doorn

contents

before you begin

Before you dive in, I want to say something clearly.

This is not homework.

You are not being graded and there's no gold star for finishing every page. You don't have to answer every question, and you definitely don't have to sound wise or put-together while you do it.

This guide exists because reading something and actually letting it sink in are two different things. Sometimes we nod along and think, "Yes, that's me," and then we close the book and move on with our day. This is just a space to pause a little longer.

Some questions will feel easy. Some might make you uncomfortable. That doesn't mean you're doing it wrong. It just means you're being honest.

You can go in order, or you can flip to whatever chapter feels personal right now. You can write a few sentences or you can fill the whole page. You can come back weeks later and see if your answers have changed.

There's no right way to do this.

If something hits harder than you expected, close the book and take a deep breath. If something feels light, let it be light. Not every chapter has to be heavy to matter.

This isn't about fixing yourself. It's about understanding yourself a little better than you did yesterday.

Write what's true. Even if it's messy. *Especially* if it's messy.

You don't have to show this to anyone.

Just be honest.

— Mary

part one
diagnosis, stigma, and speaking up

This is where we untangle the beginning.

The identity shift.

The grief no one warned you about.

The shame that settled in quietly.

The myths that shaped your thinking.

The pressure to explain yourself.

Part One is about separating who you are from what you were told.

It's about noticing what you've been carrying, and deciding what doesn't belong to you anymore.

Take your time here.

you are not
your diagnosis

. . .

TAKE A BREATH.

You just read that your diagnosis is not your identity.

Now let's untangle what still feels wrapped up together.

reflect.

1. When you were first diagnosed, what story did you immediately start telling yourself?

____

2. What did you think this diagnosis meant about your worth, your body, or your future?

____

---

3. What labels have you quietly attached to yourself since then?

4. Where does shame still show up for you?

5. In what ways are you still the same person you were before diagnosis?

6. If someone described you without mentioning diabetes at all, what would they say?

be honest.

What part of yourself have you let diabetes overshadow?

____

____

____

____

____

don't skip this.

If diabetes disappeared tomorrow, what parts of your personality, habits, or struggles would still be there?

____

____

____

____

____

what landed?

What sentence or idea from this chapter felt personal? Why do you think it hit?

____

____

____

____

____

Mary Van Doorn

your thoughts.

No fixing. No performing. Just you.

keep writing.

If your diagnosis is a chapter, what other chapters in your life deserve more attention right now?

____
____
____
____
____
____
____
____
____
____
____
____
____
____
____
____
____
____
____
____
____
____
____
____

keep writing.

grieving the life you thought you'd have

. . .

SIT WITH THIS FOR A MINUTE.

Grief doesn't only show up when you lose a person. Sometimes it shows up when life doesn't look the way you imagined.

reflect.

1. When you picture the version of your life you thought you'd have, what feels most different now?

____

____

____

____

____

2. What did you assume would feel easier by this point in your life?

____

____

____

____

____

3. Have there been moments when you felt like you "should be over this by now"?

____

____

____

____

____

4. What parts of your old routines, identity, or sense of control do you miss?

____

____

____

____

____

5. When grief shows up for you, how does it usually feel? Quiet? Angry? Heavy? Numb?

____

____

____

____

---

6. Have you been minimizing your sadness by calling it frustration, guilt, or "just a bad day"?

---

be honest.

What have you lost that you haven't fully allowed yourself to name?

---

don't rush this.

Is there pressure in your life to "stay positive" or "move on"?
How has that affected the way you process your emotions?

---

what felt uncomfortably true?

Was there a line in this chapter that made you pause? What about it felt personal?

---

your thoughts.

You don't have to tie this up neatly.

keep writing.

If you gave yourself full permission to grieve without guilt, what might change?

the stigma problem
(and why it's not you)

. . .

THIS ONE CAN STING.

Stigma doesn't always shout. Sometimes it's quiet, persistent, and personal.

reflect.

1. What messages have you heard about type 2 diabetes from media, doctors, family, or strangers?

____

____

____

____

____

2. Which of those messages did you absorb as truth about yourself?

____

____

____

____

____

3. Have you ever felt blamed or judged because of your diagnosis?
What did that moment feel like?

____

____

____

____

____

4. In what ways have you judged yourself using the same language
you've heard from others?

____

____

____

____

____

5. What assumptions do you worry people make about you?

____

____

____

____

____

. . .

6. How has stigma shaped the way you talk to yourself?

____
____
____
____
____

be honest.

Where are you still carrying shame that never actually belonged
to you?

____
____
____
____
____

don't look away.

If stigma wasn't part of the picture, how differently might you see your
diagnosis?

____
____
____
____
____

what felt personal?

Was there a moment in this chapter where you felt exposed or seen?
Why do you think it landed that way?

____

____

____

____

____

Mary Van Doorn

your thoughts.

You don't have to defend yourself here.

keep writing.

If you stopped treating diabetes like a moral report card, what would change?

but i don't look sick

. . .

INVISIBLE DOESN'T MEAN IMAGINARY.
Not all struggles show up on the outside.

reflect.

1. Have you ever felt like you had to prove your diagnosis to someone?

____

____

____

____

____

2. What does "looking sick" mean to you?

____

____

____

____

____

3. Have you ever questioned your own experience because others minimized it?

____

____

____

____

____

4. In what situations do you feel pressure to explain your health choices?

____

____

____

____

____

5. Do you ever feel like you have to perform being "fine"?

____

____

____

____

____

6. What's the cost of constantly managing other people's perceptions?

---

be honest.

Have you ever downplayed your own experience to make other people comfortable?

---

drop the performance.

If you stopped trying to look "healthy enough" or "sick enough," what would shift? Who would you be without the performance?

---

what stayed with you?

Was there a moment in this chapter that felt validating? Why did it matter?

____

____

____

____

____

Mary Van Doorn

your thoughts.

You don't owe anyone your proof.

keep writing.

What does it look like to protect your peace, even when people don't understand?

misconceptions that deserve to die out

. . .

LET'S CLEAR THE AIR.

Some of what you've been told about type 2 diabetes is incomplete, outdated, or flat-out wrong.

reflect.

1. What's the most common advice you've heard about managing diabetes?

____

____

____

____

____

2. Which "rules" have felt unrealistic or oversimplified?

____

____
____
____
____

3. Have you ever felt like you were failing because something that "should work" didn't work for you?

____
____
____
____
____

4. What messages about weight, willpower, or discipline have stuck with you?

____
____
____
____
____

5. Is there a belief you still hold that might not actually be true?

____
____
____
____
____

be honest.

What misconception have you internalized the deepest?
Where did it come from?

____
____
____
____
____

call it out.

If you could publicly correct one myth about type 2 diabetes, what
would you say?

____
____
____
____
____

what hit differently?

Did anything in this chapter challenge something you used to believe?
What shifted?

____
____
____
____
____

your thoughts.

You're allowed to question what you were taught.

Mary Van Doorn

keep writing.

What feels truer for you now?

advocacy starts with you

. . .

ADVOCACY DOESN'T HAVE **to be loud.**

Sometimes it starts with one honest sentence.

reflect.

1. Do you feel comfortable asking questions at medical appointments? Why or why not?

____
____
____
____
____

2. Have you ever left an appointment wishing you had said something?

____

____

____

____

____

3. In what areas of your health do you feel confident speaking up?

____

____

____

____

____

4. In what areas do you hesitate?

____

____

____

____

____

5. What makes it hard to advocate for yourself?

____

____

____

____

____

be honest.

Where have you stayed quiet to avoid being seen as difficult?

____

____

____

____

____

say it clearly.

If you trusted your voice completely, what would you say more often?

____

____

____

____

____

what felt empowering?

Was there a moment in this chapter that made you feel stronger or more capable? What was it?

____

____

____

____

____

your thoughts.

You are allowed to take up space in your own care.

keep writing.

What do you need people to understand about your health?
Write it the way you would say it if you weren't worried about how it would be perceived.

rethinking your
treatment plan

. . .

PLANS ARE MEANT TO EVOLVE.
Your body changes. Your life changes. Your care can change too.

reflect.

1. When was the last time you reviewed your treatment plan with curiosity instead of judgment?

____

____

____

____

____

2. Does your current plan feel supportive, overwhelming, confusing, or outdated?

____

____

____

____

____

3. Are there parts of your care that feel like obligation instead of intention?

____

____

____

____

____

4. Have you ever hesitated to ask about changing medication, adjusting doses, or trying something new?

____

____

____

____

____

5. Where do you feel confident in your management? Where do you feel stuck?

____

____

____

____

---

be honest.

Are you trying to force a plan that worked for an older version of you?

____
____
____
____
____

look at this clearly.

If your numbers aren't improving, what story are you telling yourself about why? Is it a moral story? Or a physiological one?

____
____
____
____
____

what shifted?

Did this chapter change how you see adjustments, medication, or asking for help? What felt freeing?

____
____
____
____
____

your thoughts.

Your care is allowed to grow with you.

keep writing.

If you approached your treatment plan like a partnership instead of a
test, what would that look like?

____
____
____
____
____
____
____
____
____
____
____
____
____
____
____
____
____
____
____
____
____
____
____
____
____

explaining type 2 to the world

. . .

YOU DON'T OWE **everyone an explanation.**

But sometimes explaining feels easier than being misunderstood.

reflect.

1. Who in your life knows the full truth about your diagnosis?

____

____

____

____

____

2. Who only knows parts of it?

____

____

____

____

____

42

3. Have you ever over-explained your health choices to avoid judgment?

____

____

____

____

____

4. Have you ever avoided sharing to protect your peace?

____

____

____

____

____

5. What kinds of comments trigger the urge to defend yourself?

____

____

____

____

____

6. When you explain your diagnosis, does it feel empowering or exhausting?

---

be honest.

Are you educating others because you want to…or because you feel like you have to?

---

choose this intentionally.

If you could decide who gets access to your story, who would you include? Who might not need as much detail?

---

what felt familiar?

Was there a moment in this chapter that felt like your experience?
What made it resonate?

____
____
____
____
____

your thoughts.

You get to decide how much of your story you share.

keep writing.

If you had one simple explanation ready…something calm, clear, and grounded, what would it sound like? Write it in your own words.

remission vs. reversal vs. reality

. . .

HOPE IS POWERFUL. **So is honesty.**

Not every journey looks the same. Not every outcome defines your effort.

reflect.

1. When you hear the words "remission" or "reversal," what emotions come up for you?

____

____

____

____

____

2. Have you ever compared your progress to someone else's story?

____

____

____

____

____

3. Do you feel pressure to "win" at diabetes?

____

____

____

____

____

4. What does success look like to you right now?

____

____

____

____

____

5. Have your goals shifted over time?

____

____

____

____

____

6. What feels realistic for your body and your life today?

____

____

____

____

____

be honest.

Are you chasing someone else's definition of success?

____

____

____

____

____

sit with this.

If remission never becomes your story, does that make your effort less meaningful? Why or why not?

____

____

____

____

____

what felt grounding?

Was there a moment in this chapter that made you exhale?What about
it felt stabilizing?

____
____
____
____
____

your thoughts.

Your journey is not a competition.

Mary Van Doorn

keep writing.

What does living well, not perfectly, look like for you?

part two
mindset shifts
and mental health

This is where we look at what keeps repeating.

The fear that hides behind procrastination.

The comfort of staying stuck.

The pressure to be perfect.

The comparison that steals your confidence.

The burnout you keep pushing through.

Part Two is not about blaming yourself.

It's about understanding your patterns well enough to change them.

This is where awareness turns into ownership.

Stay honest.

the fear of success
(yes, it's real)

. . .

THIS ONE HIDES **in plain sight.**

Sometimes what we call "lack of motivation" is something deeper.

reflect.

1. Have you ever made progress and then quietly pulled back?

____

____

____

____

____

2. What changes in your life when you start succeeding?

____

____

____

____

____

56

3. Who might react differently if you stepped fully into your potential?

____

____

____

____

____

4. Does success feel safe to you? Why or why not?

____

____

____

____

____

5. What part of you benefits from staying where you are?

____

____

____

____

____

be honest.

What are you afraid would happen if things actually worked?

____

____

____

____

____

look closer.

If you reached your goal, who would you have to become? Does that version of you feel exciting…or uncomfortable?

____

____

____

____

____

what felt uncomfortably true?

Was there a moment in this chapter that sounded like something you've done before? What did you recognize?

____

____

____

____

____

your thoughts.

No judgment. Just patterns.

keep writing.

If you stopped shrinking right before momentum builds, what might be possible?

comfort zones, chaos, and why getting stuck makes sense

. . .

STUCK ISN'T ALWAYS LAZINESS.
Sometimes it's protection.

reflect.

1. When you think about real change, what feels most uncomfortable?

____
____
____
____
____

2. Is there a version of "stuck" that feels strangely familiar or predictable?

____
____

____

____

____

3. Have you ever chosen chaos because at least you knew how to manage it?

____

____

____

____

____

4. What patterns do you repeat, even when you know they don't serve you?

____

____

____

____

____

5. Does calm progress ever feel boring compared to urgency or drama?

____

____

____

____

____

be honest.

What are you protecting by staying where you are?

____
____
____
____
____

look closer.

If getting unstuck meant stepping into unfamiliar territory, what would that require from you? Courage? Vulnerability? Consistency?

____
____
____
____
____

what felt personal?

Did anything in this chapter sound like your own behavior? What did you recognize?

____
____
____
____
____

your thoughts.

Familiar doesn't always mean healthy.

keep writing.

If chaos feels normal, what would "stable" feel like in your life?

the emotional
weight of weight loss

. . .

CHANGE **on the outside doesn't automatically settle the inside.**

reflect.

1. How has your relationship with your body changed over the years?

____

____

____

____

____

2. Have people treated you differently based on your weight? What did that feel like?

____

____

____

____

____

3. Did weight loss bring what you expected? What surprised you?

____

____

____

____

____

4. Have you ever felt pressure to maintain a specific version of yourself?

____

____

____

____

____

5. When your body changes, does your sense of worth shift with it?

____

____

____

____

____

6. Is there grief attached to any version of your body, past or present?

\
\
\
\
\

be honest.

Has weight loss ever felt like proof that you were finally "doing it right"? What happens to your self-talk when the scale doesn't cooperate?

\
\
\
\
\

look deeper.

If your body changed again tomorrow, who would you be without the reaction from others?

\
\
\
\
\

what felt complicated?

Was there a part of this chapter that disrupted the idea that weight loss fixes everything? What did it stir up?

____
____
____
____
____

your thoughts.

Progress is allowed to be complex.

Mary Van Doorn

keep writing.

What does self-worth look like when it isn't tied to your size?

from burnout
to boundaries

· · ·

YOU CAN'T POUR **from an empty cup.**
And you don't have to earn rest.

reflect.

1. What does burnout look like for you — physically or emotionally?

____

____

____

____

____

2. Do you tend to push through exhaustion instead of acknowledging it?

____

____

____

____

____

3. Where in your life do you feel over-responsible?

____

____

____

____

____

4. Are there expectations you've accepted without questioning?

____

____

____

____

____

5. When was the last time you rested without guilt?

____

____

____

____

____

6. What drains you the fastest: people, decisions, perfection, constant monitoring?

____

____

____

____

____

be honest.

Are you tired because of your workload…or because of your lack of boundaries?

____

____

____

____

____

say it clearly.

Where do you need a boundary, even if it feels uncomfortable to set one?

____

____

____

____

____

what hit close to home?

Was there a moment in this chapter that made you realize you've been running on empty? What did you recognize?

____

____

____

____

____

your thoughts.

Rest is not a reward.

keep writing.

If you treated your energy like something valuable and limited, what would change?

the perfectionism trap

. . .

PERFECTION FEELS PRODUCTIVE. **Until it isn't.**

reflect.

1. Where does perfectionism show up most in your life?

____
____
____
____
____

2. Do you tend to start strong and then quit when things aren't perfect?

____
____
____
____

3. What does "doing it right" mean to you?

4. How do you talk to yourself when you fall short of your own expectations?

5. Have you ever delayed action because you were waiting for the perfect plan?

6. What happens to your motivation when you make one mistake?

____

____

____

____

be honest.

Is perfection protecting you from something? What would happen if you were just consistent instead of perfect?

____

____

____

____

____

look closer.

Who taught you that effort only counts if it's flawless? Is that belief still serving you?

____

____

____

____

____

what felt familiar?

Did you recognize your own patterns in this chapter? Where do you see them most clearly?

your thoughts.

Done imperfectly still counts.

keep writing.

If you allowed yourself to be messy and steady instead of perfect and extreme, what might change?

comparison is a confidence killer

. . .

IT'S hard to feel steady when you're constantly measuring.

reflect.

1. Who do you tend to compare yourself to?

____

____

____

____

____

2. What specifically do you compare: weight, numbers, discipline, speed of progress?

____

____

____

____

____

3. How does comparison affect your motivation?

____

____

____

____

____

4. Does it make you push harder…or shut down?

____

____

____

____

____

5. Have you ever felt "behind" because someone else's story moved faster?

____

____

____

____

____

6. What do you assume about people whose outcomes look better than yours?

____

____

____

____

____

be honest.

When you compare yourself to others, what are you really looking for? Validation? Proof? Permission?

____

____

____

____

____

look at this clearly.

If you stopped using someone else's timeline as your benchmark, what would success look like for you?

____

____

____

____

____

what felt exposed?

Was there a moment in this chapter that made you realize comparison has been louder than you thought? What did you notice?

____

____

____

____

____

your thoughts.

Your pace is not a competition.

keep writing.

If you trusted your own timeline, what would change about the way you show up?

motivation is a liar (and why you don't need it)

. . .

FEELINGS ARE UNRELIABLE. **Action is not.**

reflect.

1. How often do you wait to "feel motivated" before you start
something?

____

____

____

____

____

2. What does motivation feel like to you?

____

____

____

---

3. When motivation fades, what usually happens next?

---

4. Have you ever mistaken lack of motivation for lack of ability?

---

5. What habits have you built even when you didn't feel like it?

6. Do you believe you need to feel inspired to be consistent?

____

____

____

____

____

be honest.

Are you using motivation as permission to delay action?

____

____

____

____

____

look closer.

If you stopped waiting to feel ready, what would you do differently this week?

____

____

____

____

____

what felt challenging?

Was there a moment in this chapter that disrupted how you think about discipline or consistency? What shifted?

your thoughts.

You don't need hype to move.

keep writing.

If consistency mattered more than intensity, what would your next step look like?

visualization, vibes,
and victory laps

. . .

YOU DON'T ONLY HAVE **to fix what's wrong.**
You're allowed to picture what's possible.

reflect.

1. When you imagine a version of yourself who feels steady and strong, what does that look like?

____

____

____

____

____

2. Do you allow yourself to celebrate small progress, or do you move the goalpost?

____

---

3. What would it feel like to acknowledge your wins more often?

---

4. When was the last time you paused long enough to notice growth?

---

lean into this.

If you believed change was possible for you, what would you picture?

---

what felt energizing?

Was there a moment in this chapter that made you feel hopeful? What stood out?

____

____

____

____

____

Mary Van Doorn

your thoughts.

Progress deserves to be noticed.

keep writing.

What is one win, small or big, that you haven't fully given yourself credit for?

the mindset shift that changed everything

. . .

THIS ISN'T **about doing more.**

It's about thinking differently so you stop starting over from the same place.

reflect.

1. What belief about yourself has shaped your health choices the most?

____

____

____

____

____

2. Have you ever changed your behavior without changing your thinking?

____

____

____

____

____

3. What thought pattern shows up most during setbacks?

____

____

____

____

____

4. When you struggle, what story do you default to?

____

____

____

____

____

5. Is there a mindset you've outgrown, but still operate from?

____

____

____

____

____

be honest.

What belief about yourself needs to change for progress to stick?

____

____

____

____

____

look at this clearly.

If you stopped seeing yourself as someone who "always struggles," who would you become?

____

____

____

____

____

what clicked?

Was there a moment in this chapter where something felt obvious in a new way? What shifted?

____

____

____

____

____

your thoughts.

Thoughts create direction.

keep writing.

If one mindset shift could change your trajectory over the next year, what would it be?

taking the long way home

. . .

QUICK FIXES FEEL EXCITING.
Slow growth lasts longer.

reflect.

1. Have you ever chased fast results over sustainable change?

____

____

____

____

____

2. What does "slow progress" feel like to you?

____

____

____

---

3. Do you get impatient when results don't come quickly?

---

4. Where in your life have you seen steady effort pay off?

---

5. What makes long-term thinking hard for you?

be honest.

Are you trying to sprint through something that requires endurance?

____

____

____

____

____

look at this clearly.

If this journey takes longer than you hoped, does that make it less worth it?

____

____

____

____

____

what felt grounding?

Was there a part of this chapter that made you exhale? What about it steadied you?

____

____

____

____

____

your thoughts.

There is no rush.

keep writing.

If you committed to the long way, imperfect, steady, and patient, what would that look like?

your why (and how to find it again)

. . .

YOUR WHY ISN'T GONE.
It might just be buried under exhaustion or distraction.

reflect.

1. When you first started taking your health seriously, what mattered most to you?

____

____

____

____

____

2. Has your why changed over time?

____

____

____

____

____

3. What originally motivated you that no longer feels strong?

____

____

____

____

____

4. When you feel disconnected from your goals, what's usually happening in your life?

____

____

____

____

____

5. Do your current habits reflect what you say matters to you?

____

____

____

____

____

be honest.

Is your why truly yours…or something you think it should be?

____

____

____

____

____

look closer.

If no one else's expectations existed, what would matter most about your health?

____

____

____

____

____

what felt personal?

Was there a moment in this chapter that reminded you of something you'd forgotten? What was it?

____

____

____

____

____

your thoughts.

Clarity fuels consistency.

keep writing.

If you reconnected to your why in a quiet, steady way, not dramatic, or urgent, what would shift?

healing from setbacks
without starting over

. . .

A SETBACK ISN'T A RESET.
It's a moment. Not a verdict.

reflect.

1. When you experience a setback, what is your first internal reaction?

____

____

____

____

____

2. Do you tend to see missteps as failure or information?

____

____

____

____

____

3. How long do you usually stay stuck after something goes "off plan"?

____

____

____

____

____

4. What story do you tell yourself in the middle of a setback?

____

____

____

____

____

5. Have you ever made one mistake mean something bigger about who you are?

____

____

____

____

____

be honest.

Do you use setbacks as permission to quit?

____

____

____

____

____

look at this clearly.

If you stopped starting over every time you slipped, what would change about your progress?

____

____

____

____

____

what felt stabilizing?

Was there a moment in this chapter that helped you see setbacks differently? What shifted?

____

____

____

____

____

your thoughts.

Progress doesn't disappear.

keep writing.

If you treated setbacks as part of the process instead of proof you failed, how would you move forward?

____

____

____

____

____

____

____

____

____

____

____

____

____

____

____

____

____

____

____

____

____

____

____

____

journaling
without eye rolls

. . .

THIS ISN'T **about being poetic.**
It's about being honest on paper.

reflect.

1. What comes to mind when you hear the word "journaling"?

____

____

____

____

____

2. Have you ever tried it and quit? Why?

____

____

____

____

____

3. Do you think your thoughts are clearer in your head…or once they're written down?

____

____

____

____

____

4. When your mind feels crowded, what usually happens next?

____

____

____

____

____

5. What would make journaling feel less forced and more useful?

____

____

____

____

____

be honest.

Are you avoiding writing things down because you don't want to see them clearly?

---

try this differently.

If journaling was simply a brain dump, not a performance, what would you write?

---

what felt doable?

Was there something in this chapter that made journaling feel less intimidating? What shifted?

---

your thoughts.

Messy is allowed.

keep writing.

Write whatever is on your mind right now. No structure. No filter. Just start.

part three
habits, healing, and everyday wins

This is where it gets lived out.

Not perfectly.

Not dramatically.

Not all at once.

Part Three is about what happens on regular days.

The choices you make when no one is watching.

The habits that feel small but add up.

This is where mindset becomes movement.

Not extreme.

Not urgent.

Just steady.

Keep it simple.

food is not a moral test

. . .

EATING IS NOT A REPORT CARD.
It's information.

reflect.

1. What foods still trigger guilt for you?

____

____

____

____

____

2. When you label a food as "bad," what story follows?

____

____

____

____

____

3. How does judgment change the way you eat?

____

____

____

____

____

notice the pattern.

When you feel guilt around food, what usually happens next? Restriction? Overeating? Giving up?

____

____

____

____

____

try this.

For one week, remove moral language from your food choices.
Instead of:
"I was bad."
Try:
"That choice didn't align with how I want to feel."
Write down what shifts when you change the wording.

Mary Van Doorn

your thoughts.

Neutral is powerful.

small step.

What is one meal this week where you can practice curiosity instead of criticism?

____

small step.

your plate, your plan

. . .

THERE ISN'T **one right way.**
There's the way that works for you.

reflect.

1. Have you ever followed a plan that worked for someone else but not for you?

____
____
____
____
____

2. What makes a plan feel sustainable in your real life?

____
____

---

3. What tends to derail you: complexity, restriction, boredom?

---

quick inventory.

Circle what matters most in your current season:
- Simplicity
- Structure
- Flexibility
- Accountability
- Variety
- Convenience
- Cost
- Family-friendly
- Low mental load

What stands out?

---

experiment.

If you simplified your eating plan by 20 percent this week, what would you remove? What would you keep?

____

____

____

____

____

your thoughts.

Your life determines your plan.

Mary Van Doorn

this week.

Choose one small adjustment that makes your plan feel more doable, not more perfect.

diet culture detox

. . .

SOME OF WHAT **you believe about food was taught to you.**
That doesn't mean you have to keep it.

reflect.

1. What messages about food and weight did you grow up hearing?

____

____

____

____

____

2. Which of those messages still influence how you eat today?

____

____

____

---

3. Do you believe health has to look a certain way?

---

notice this.

When you feel guilt around food, whose voice does it sound like?
Is it yours? A parent? A coach? A diet plan?

---

experiment.

For the next week, question one rule you've always accepted.
Example:
"I can't eat after 7."
"I shouldn't eat carbs."
"I have to earn dessert."
Ask:
Is this serving me right now?

Write down what you discover.

____

____

____

____

____

your thoughts.

Unlearning takes patience.

small step.

What is one belief about food you are ready to loosen your grip on?

accountability, not isolation

. . .

YOU ARE **responsible for your choices.**
But you don't have to carry them alone.

reflect.

1. When you struggle, do you tend to withdraw or reach out?

____

____

____

____

____

2. What does accountability mean to you?

____

____

____

____

____

3. Have you ever confused isolation with independence?

____

____

____

____

____

notice this.

When no one knows your goals, how does that affect your follow-through? When someone does know, what changes?

____

____

____

____

____

practice this.

Choose one person you trust and share one specific goal with them.
Not for pressure.
For support.

Write down how it feels to say it out loud.

____
____
____
____
____

your thoughts.

Connection strengthens commitment.

Mary Van Doorn

this week.

What is one small way you can stay visible instead of going silent?

support systems: building
a circle that holds you up

. . .

SUPPORT ISN'T **about having people around you.**
It's about having people who show up.

reflect.

1. Who in your life feels safe to be honest with?

____

____

____

____

____

2. Who encourages you without policing you?

____

____

____

---

3. Where do you feel supported right now, even in small ways?

---

quick inventory.

Think about the people around you. Who tends to:
• Listen without fixing
• Celebrate your wins
• Respect your boundaries
• Check in consistently
• Show up when it matters

Write down the names that come to mind.

---

build intentionally.

If your circle feels small, what's one place you could expand it?
A group? A class? A conversation you've avoided?

____

____

____

____

____

Mary Van Doorn

your thoughts.

Support is built, not stumbled into.

small step.

Reach out to one person this week, not to vent, but to connect.

when support
systems suck

. . .

NOT EVERYONE WILL GET IT.
That doesn't make your needs unreasonable.

reflect.

1. Have you ever felt dismissed or misunderstood about your health?

____

____

____

____

____

2. Do certain people make your goals harder instead of easier?

____

____

____

---

3. Have you minimized your own needs to avoid conflict?

notice this.

When someone questions your choices, how do you usually respond? Silence? Defense? Humor? Withdrawal?

---

protect your energy.

If someone consistently undermines your progress, what boundary might be necessary? It doesn't have to be dramatic. Just clear.

---

this week.

What is one sentence you could practice that honors your boundary?

____

____

____

____

____

your thoughts.

You are allowed to protect your peace.

why you keep quitting and how to quit that

. . .

QUITTING USUALLY FOLLOWS A PATTERN.
So does staying.

reflect.

1. When you've quit before, what happened right before that decision?

____

____

____

____

____

2. Do you tend to quit after a mistake, boredom, overwhelm, or slow progress?

____

____

____

____

____

3. What story do you tell yourself when things feel hard?

____

____

____

____

____

spot the cycle.

Write out your usual pattern:
Start →
Momentum →
Trigger →
Reaction →
Quit

What's the trigger most often?

____

____

____

____

____

change one link.

Instead of trying to "never quit again," what if you only interrupted one part of the cycle? Which part feels most doable to adjust?

____

____

____

____

____

Mary Van Doorn

your thoughts.

Patterns can be rewritten.

this week.

When you feel the urge to quit, pause for 24 hours before deciding anything. Write down what changes when you delay the decision.

goal setting that doesn't suck

. . .

GOALS SHOULDN'T FEEL **like punishment.**
They should feel possible.

reflect.

1. When you think about setting goals, what emotion comes up first?

____
____
____
____
____

2. Do your goals usually feel motivating or overwhelming?

____
____
____

---

3. Have you ever set a goal you thought you "should" want?

---

4. What makes a goal feel heavy instead of helpful?

---

rethink this.

If a goal feels exhausting before you even begin, what might that be telling you? Too big? Too vague? Not actually yours?

Mary Van Doorn

simplify.

Instead of asking, "What's my big goal?"
Ask, "What feels important right now?"
Write down one focus for this season…not forever. Just for now.

____
____
____
____
____

your thoughts.

Small is not insignificant.

this week.

What is one action that supports your focus without requiring perfection?

the power of one thing

. . .

YOU DON'T NEED **to fix everything at once.**

You just need one thing you'll actually follow through on.

reflect.

1. When you try to change too many things at once, what usually happens?

____
____
____
____
____

2. Do you feel more motivated by big overhauls or small shifts?

____
____

---

3. What is one area of your health that would make everything else feel easier if it improved?

---

narrow it down.

If you could only focus on one habit for the next 30 days, what would it be? Not the most impressive one, the most doable one.

---

simplify.

What makes that one thing realistic in your current season?
What would make it unnecessarily complicated?

---

your thoughts.

Focused effort builds momentum.

this week.

Write your one thing below. Then write the smallest version of it you're willing to commit to.

movement that works for you

. . .

MOVEMENT DOESN'T HAVE to be extreme to be effective.
It just has to be consistent.

reflect.

1. What kind of movement have you enjoyed at any point in your life?

____

____

____

____

____

2. What kind of movement have you forced yourself to do because you thought you should?

____

____

____
____
____

3. When you skip workouts, what's usually the reason — time, energy, intimidation, boredom?

____
____
____
____
____

4. Do you associate exercise with punishment or progress?

____
____
____
____
____

shift this.

If movement was about feeling stronger, not smaller, what would change?

____
____
____
____
____

simplify.

Instead of asking, "What workout should I do?"
Ask, "What can I do today that moves my body?"
Walk. Stretch. Lift. Dance. Clean. Play.

Write down three options that feel realistic in your current season.

____

____

____

____

____

Mary Van Doorn

your thoughts.

Movement is a tool, not a test.

this week.

Pick one type of movement that feels doable and commit to it...not perfectly, just consistently.

this week.

redefining wellness (and what self-care actually is)
. . .

WELLNESS ISN'T A VIBE.
It's how you take care of yourself when life is full.

reflect.

1. When you hear "self-care," what comes to mind?

____
____
____
____
____

2. Is your version of wellness realistic for your current season of life?

____

____

____

____

____

3. Do you treat self-care as a reward or a responsibility?

____

____

____

____

____

4. Where are you neglecting your own capacity?

____

____

____

____

____

look at this differently.

If self-care meant preserving your health instead of indulging yourself, what would that include? Sleep? Boundaries? Medication? Saying no?

____

____

____

____

____

Mary Van Doorn

redefine it.

Write your own definition of wellness right now…not the aspirational version. The livable one.

____
____
____
____
____

your thoughts.

Sustainable beats impressive.

this week.

What is one form of self-care that protects your energy instead of just distracting you?

celebrating progress, not just results

. . .

RESULTS ARE VISIBLE.
Progress often isn't.

reflect.

1. What changes have you made that no one else can see?

____

____

____

____

____

2. How has your thinking shifted over the past year?

____

____

____

____

____

3. Where are you more consistent than you used to be?

____

____

____

____

____

4. What effort have you overlooked because the outcome wasn't
dramatic?

____

____

____

____

____

pause here.

If you measured growth by effort instead of outcome, what would you
notice?

____

____

____

____

____

look back.

Think about where you were when you first started this journey. What feels different now, even slightly?

____

____

____

____

____

Mary Van Doorn

your thoughts.

Small shifts count.

keep this.

Write down three ways you have grown that have nothing to do with
the scale.

____

____

____

____

____

____

____

____

____

____

____

____

____

____

____

____

____

____

____

____

____

____

keep this.

wrapping it up

If you've made it this far, that tells me something about you.

You're willing to look at yourself honestly. You're willing to sit with discomfort. You're willing to try again instead of pretending you don't care.

That's not small.

Some of these pages might feel clear and complete. Others might feel messy. You might have skipped a question. You might have written more than you expected. That's how this is supposed to work.

This wasn't about answering everything perfectly. It was about noticing what's true for you.

Maybe you uncovered patterns you hadn't noticed before.

Maybe you softened the way you talk to yourself.

Maybe you realized you've been carrying more than you needed to.

Whatever shifted, even slightly, counts.

You don't need a dramatic transformation to call this progress. Sometimes the win is simply not quitting on yourself.

Close this book knowing you are more aware than you were. More steady than you think. More capable than you give yourself credit for.

You are allowed to ask questions.

Wrapping it Up

You are allowed to take up space in your care.
You are allowed to trust your own judgment.
That's confidence.
And you're not done.

Keep going.